Your Anger Is Valid

If Only You Can Rise Above Rage

7 practical steps Women can tame rage and manage anger

By Flor Bentley

Content

Preface

My Journey to Managing Anger

I always prided myself on being a caring and dedicated mother, but i found myself increasingly losing my temper over small things. The constant stress of balancing work, family, and personal expectations was taking its toll. One evening, after an argument with my teenage daughter over a missed curfew, i realized i needed to make a change.

I started by reading some books, and meditating which helped me understand that my anger was a valid emotion, but how i expressed it needed to be worked on. I began practicing mindfulness and deep breathing exercises, learning to pause and breathe before reacting. I also started journaling, identifying my triggers, and recognizing the physical signs of anger building up.

I was able to attend an anger management workshop and built a supportive network of friends who understood my struggles. I learned to set boundaries and communicate my needs assertively without yelling. Slowly but surely, i began to notice some change, I felt more in control, my outbursts became less frequent, and my relationship with my daughter improved significantly.

Now, i feel empowered and proud of my journey. The techniques i learned and practiced to maintain my emotional health and turn moments of potential rage into opportunities for growth and understanding are all detailed in this book with practical steps to follow.

You need to grab a cup of coffee, tea, or wine to sip from occasionally as you read through to gain more insight on how to manage anger and rise above rage.

Introduction

Welcome and Purpose

Welcome

Welcome to "Your Anger is Valid: If Only You Can Rise Above Rage: 7 Practical Steps Women Can Tame Rage and Manage Anger." This book empowers women to understand and manage their anger constructively. Whether you experience anger frequently or occasionally, this guide is here to help you navigate and transform your relationship with this powerful emotion.

Purpose

The purpose of this book is to provide you with practical tools and strategies to manage your anger in healthy and constructive ways. When understood and channeled appropriately, anger can be a source of strength and positive change. We aim to help you harness this energy to improve your well-being and relationships.

Importance of Addressing Anger

Why Acknowledging and Managing Anger is Crucial

Anger is a normal and acceptable emotion, but when left uncontrolled, it may harm your health, relationships, and general quality of life. Here's why it's crucial to recognize and control your anger:

Personal Well-Being:

- ***Physical Health:*** Unmanaged anger may lead to several health consequences, including high blood pressure, heart disease, and a compromised immune system. Chronic anger may also lead to headaches, digestive difficulties, and sleep disruptions.
- ***Mental Health:*** Anger may raise stress levels, leading to anxiety and sadness. Addressing anger constructively may enhance your mood and mental health,

encouraging a more balanced and calm frame of mind.

Relationships:

- ***Communication:*** Anger typically leads to poor communication, misunderstandings, and relationship conflict. Learning to express anger constructively may boost your communication skills and improve your connections with others.
- ***Trust and Intimacy:*** Consistently expressing anger in negative ways may erode trust and closeness in relationships. By regulating your anger, you may develop deeper, more trustworthy ties with family, friends, and coworkers.

Self-Esteem and Empowerment:

- ***Self-Respect:*** Managing anger correctly helps you preserve self-respect and dignity. It permits you to stand up for yourself without resorting to harsh or damaging activities.

- ***Empowerment:*** Taking control of your anger allows you to make great changes in your life. It supports your capacity to manage hard circumstances with elegance and perseverance.

Social and Professional Life:

- ***Conflict Resolution:*** Developing anger management skills may boost your capacity to settle disagreements constructively, leading to more harmonious social and professional relationships.
- ***Job Advancement:*** Effective anger control may enhance your work connections and reputation, perhaps leading to improved job prospects and success.

Moving Forward

Throughout this book, you will discover practical strategies, contemplative activities, and helpful resources to help you understand and control your anger. By committing to this journey, you are taking a huge step towards personal development and healthy relationships. Remember, your anger is real, and with the correct skills, you can rise beyond wrath to lead a more powerful and fulfilled life.

Let's begin this transformational adventure together.

Chapter 1: Understanding Anger

What exactly is anger?

Anger is a strong and multifaceted emotion that manifests itself in reaction to perceived threats, injustices, or disappointments. The intensity of this reaction may vary from moderate annoyance to violent rage, and it is a normal and instinctual response. Recognizing anger as a signal that something in your surroundings or inside yourself needs attention and resolution is an important step toward understanding anger.

Defining Anger

The level of anger may range from slight irritation to tremendous hatred and fury. Anger is a state of mind that everyone can experience. As is the case with other feelings, it is accompanied by physiological and biological changes. For example, when you get furious, your heart rate and blood pressure increase, as do the levels of your energy hormones adrenaline and noradrenaline. Both internal and external occurrences have the potential to bring up anger. You might be furious at a particular person (such as a colleague or boss) or an incident (traffic congestion, a canceled trip), or your anger could be induced by fretting or brooding about your concerns. In addition, memories of traumatic or upsetting situations have the potential to bring up feelings of anger.

Comparison of Healthy and Unhealthy Ways to Express Anger

Healthy Expressions of Anger

Assertive Communication: Clearly and politely express your emotions and needs without being aggressive or passive. This may lead to problem-solving and resolution.

Physical Activity: Engage in exercise or physical activity to release built-up energy and alleviate stress.

Time-Outs: Pause a hot situation to calm down and collect your thoughts before replying.

Seeking Support: Talk to a trustworthy friend, family member, or therapist about what is making you furious.

Mindfulness and Relaxation: Practice mindfulness, deep breathing, or relaxation methods to help quiet your mind and body.

Unhealthy Expressions of Anger

Aggression: Reacting forcefully or aggressively towards others, which might involve physical aggression, yelling, or verbal abuse. This style of expression may disrupt relationships and lead to bad outcomes.

Passive-Aggression: Indirectly showing anger via actions like sarcasm, procrastination, or being morose. This may produce misunderstanding and irritation in relationships.

Suppression: Holding in anger and not expressing it, which may lead to emotional tension, resentment, and physical health difficulties such as high blood pressure or depression.

Self-Harm: Turning rage inward and injuring oneself physically or mentally. This is a risky and unhealthy method to manage anger.

Destructive Behaviors: Engaging in behaviors that are detrimental to oneself or others, such as drug misuse or reckless driving, as a means to deal with anger.

To learn how to control your anger, you must first identify the good and bad ways to show it. While there are good and bad ways to express anger, the former may help you grow while the latter can hurt your relationships and overall health. You can channel this intense feeling into something positive through the change in your life if you learn to recognize and practice healthy methods to express anger.

Chapter 2: Validating Your Anger

Acceptance

Anger is a normal, human feeling that everyone goes through at some point in their lives. In circumstances in which we feel threatened, mistreated, or irritated, it is a natural and appropriate response to have this reaction. A purpose is served by rage, just as it is by pleasure, sorrow, or fear. It notifies us of problems that demand our attention and has the potential to inspire us to make adjustments or to safeguard ourselves at the same time.

The first step toward properly controlling anger is to acknowledge that it is a rational emotion. By embracing your anger, you admit that your sentiments are genuine and deserve to be acknowledged and understood. This affirmation is vital because it enables you to not disregard or conceal your feelings, which may lead to more major concerns over time, such as chronic stress, anxiety, or depression.

When you embrace your anger, you permit yourself to experience it without judgment. This acceptance helps you to investigate the underlying reasons for your anger, recognize your needs and limits, and develop constructive methods to confront the events that elicit these sentiments.

Challenging Guilt

Many women feel guilty about expressing anger owing to cultural expectations that they should always be loving, calm, and agreeable. This guilt might arise from societal standards, upbringing, or personal views that classify rage as a bad or inappropriate feeling, particularly for women.

Challenging this guilt is vital for your mental wellness. Feeling guilty about your anger typically leads to repressing or dismissing your feelings, which may result in unresolved anger emerging in harmful ways. It's crucial to remember that getting furious does not make you a horrible person. Instead, it implies that something in your life needs to be addressed.

To Combat Guilt Effectively

- ***Acknowledge Your Emotions:*** Accept that it is acceptable to be furious. Emotions are normal reactions to our experiences, and rage is a reasonable indicator that something is not right.

- ***Reframe Negative thoughts:*** Identify and question any negative thoughts you have about anger. Understand that rage, when addressed properly, can be a beneficial force for transformation and personal progress.

- ***Self-compassion:*** Treat oneself with love and understanding. Recognize that everyone experiences anger and that it is a part of being human. Practice self-compassion by reminding yourself that it is appropriate to feel and express rage.

- ***Validate Your Experiences:*** Understand the exact causes behind your rage. Validate your emotions by addressing the events or acts that provoked your anger and why they are significant to you.

- ***Vent Anger Constructively:*** Find healthy methods to vent your anger, such as talking to a trusted friend, writing in a diary, or participating in physical exercise. Constructive expression helps to discharge pent-up emotions without causing damage to yourself or others.

By addressing the guilt linked to anger and recognizing your feelings, you may better understand and control your anger. This technique helps you turn anger into a positive force, helping you to establish boundaries, advocate for yourself, and make essential adjustments in your life. Remember, your anger is legitimate, and recognizing it is a key step toward emotional health and empowerment.

Chapter 3: The Impact of Uncontrolled Anger

Personal and Interpersonal Consequences

How Unmanaged Anger Affects Personal Well-Being

1. ***Physical Health Issues:*** Chronic anger may lead to several physical health concerns. Prolonged anger increases the body's fight-or-flight response, raising stress chemicals like adrenaline and cortisol. Over time, this may result in high blood pressure, heart disease, reduced immune system, headaches, and digestive difficulties.

2. ***Mental Health Problems:*** Unmanaged anger is often connected to mental health difficulties such as anxiety and depression. Constant anger may lead to feelings of pessimism, poor self-esteem, and chronic

tension, producing a cycle of unpleasant emotions that are hard to stop.

3. ***Impaired Judgment and Decision Making:*** When anger takes control, it may confuse your judgment and damage your decision-making ability. This emotional hijacking might lead to rash acts and choices that you may later regret.

4. ***Decreased Quality of Life:*** Persistent anger might impair your overall quality of life. It may interfere with your capacity to enjoy ordinary activities, produce a persistent feeling of unhappiness, and deprive you of inner serenity and pleasure.

How Unmanaged Anger Affects Relationships

1. ***Communication Breakdown:*** Anger typically leads to poor communication. Instead of addressing difficulties quietly, you can turn to ranting, accusing, or

condemning, which can increase tensions and inhibit fruitful interactions.

2. ***Erosion of Trust:*** Repeated outbursts of uncontrollable rage may undermine trust in relationships. Loved ones may feel uncomfortable, insulted, or underappreciated, leading to emotional distancing and loss of closeness.

3. ***Cycle of Conflict:*** Unmanaged anger may generate a cycle of conflict where unresolved concerns continually recur. This continual stress may strain relationships, making it difficult to sustain healthy and supportive ties.

4. ***Negative Impact on Children:*** For parents, unchecked anger may have harmful repercussions on children. It may create an atmosphere of dread and instability, harming children's emotional development and behavior.

Cultural and Social Context

Societal Expectations and Gender Roles Influence on Women's Anger Expression

- ***Cultural Conventions and Conditioning:*** Societal conventions frequently demand that women should be caring, docile, and accommodating. These expectations might teach women to repress their emotions and put others' demands above their own. From an early age, females are typically trained to avoid conflict and preserve peace, which may lead to internalized anger and guilt when they do feel furious.

- ***Fear of Judgment:*** Women who express rage openly are typically branded as "hysterical," "emotional," or "irrational." This fear of unfavorable evaluation may lead to self-censorship when women repress their anger to avoid being viewed as unlikable or out of control.

- ***Gender Roles in Partnerships:*** Traditional gender roles in partnerships frequently put women in caretaking and supporting roles. This dynamic may create imbalances where women's needs and emotions, especially rage, are reduced or neglected. Consequently, women could feel rejected and struggle to express their anger constructively.

- ***Workplace Dynamics:*** In professional contexts, women exhibiting anger might be considered unprofessional or excessively emotional, whereas males may be seen as aggressive or powerful for comparable conduct. This double standard might deter women from communicating their emotions and exerting themselves, resulting in untreated grievances and tension.

- ***Media Representation:*** The media typically presents angry women in a bad way, perpetuating stereotypes that restrict women from expressing anger. These depictions may impact society's views and foster the impression that women's rage is undesirable or unpleasant.

Impact of Societal Expectations on Women's Anger

- ***Suppression of Emotions:*** The pressure to adhere to societal norms might force women to repress their anger, resulting in internalized tension and emotional anguish. This suppression may appear as passive-aggressive conduct, anxiety, sadness, and other mental health concerns.

- ***Loss of Authenticity:*** Constantly suppressing their rage to match cultural conventions might make women feel distant from their genuine selves. This lack of authenticity might limit personal development and self-esteem, as women could struggle to acknowledge their own emotions and needs.

- ***Barrier to Assertiveness:*** Fear of unfavorable labels might inhibit women from being assertive and sticking up for themselves. This lack of assertiveness may lead to unresolved disputes, unmet demands, and a feeling of helplessness in personal and professional relationships.

- ***Impact on Advocacy:*** Women who repress their anger may find it hard to advocate for societal or personal reforms. Anger, when used constructively, can be a tremendous motivation for action and campaigning for justice and equality.

We can start to address and change women's angry behaviors if we acknowledge the social and cultural factors that influence their displays of anger and the emotional and interpersonal consequences of anger management issues. By teaching women to recognize and manage their anger healthily, we can improve their health and wellness and foster more equitable relationships and communities.

Chapter 4: The Power of Self-Awareness

Recognizing Triggers

Understanding what particularly causes your anger is a vital step in controlling it properly. Triggers might vary significantly from person to person, but popular ones include:

1. ***Interpersonal Conflicts:*** Arguments, conflicts, or misunderstandings with others.
2. ***Perceived Injustices:*** Feeling mistreated or treated unjustly.
3. ***tension and Overwhelm:*** High levels of tension or feeling overwhelmed with duties.
4. ***Disrespect and Criticism:*** Feeling disrespected, criticized, or not appreciated.
5. ***Personal Values and Beliefs:*** Situations that contradict your firmly held values or beliefs.
6. ***prior experiences:*** memories or reminders of prior unpleasant or distressing occurrences.

To identify your personal anger triggers:

Reflect on past experiences: Think about recent occasions when you were furious. What were the circumstances? Who was involved? What was going on around you?

Look for Patterns: Note any repeating themes or events that frequently provoke your wrath.

Consider your values: Reflect on your essential principles and beliefs. How may they impact your emotional reactions to particular situations?

Ask for Feedback: Sometimes, people might identify patterns in our behavior that we overlook. Ask trustworthy friends or family members if they've identified any unique causes for your rage.

Physical and Emotional Signals

Recognizing the early stages of anger might help you handle it before it grows. These indicators might be physical, emotional, or behavioral.

Physical Signals

- ***Increased Heart Rate:*** Feeling your heart pounding quicker.
- ***Muscle tension:*** tightness in your shoulders, neck, or jaw.
- ***Clenched Fists:*** Unconsciously gripping your hands.
- ***Feeling Hot or Flushed:*** Experiencing a burst of heat or perspiration.
- ***Stomach upset:*** feeling a knot in your stomach or nausea.

Emotional Signals

- ***Irritability:*** feeling easily irritated or on edge.
- ***Frustration:*** experiencing a sensation of frustration or impotence.
- ***Anxiety:*** feeling uneasy or apprehensive.
- ***Anger:*** harboring sentiments of anger or bitterness.

Behavioral Signals

- ***Raising Your Voice:*** Speaking louder or more fiercely.
- ***Pacing or fidgeting:*** increased physical restlessness.
- ***Interrupting:*** cutting off people in discourse.
- ***Negative Self-Talk:*** Engaging in critical or antagonistic self-talk.

Techniques For Recognition

Body Scanning: Regularly check in with your body throughout the day to discover any symptoms of tension or stress.

Mindfulness: Practice mindfulness to become more aware of your emotional state and physical experiences.

Deep Breathing: Use deep breathing techniques to quiet your body and mind, making it easier to identify small changes.

Journaling Prompts

Journaling is a fantastic technique for examining your emotions and getting insight into your anger triggers and reactions.

Here are some journaling prompts to help enhance your self-awareness:

* ***Recent Anger Experience:*** Describe a recent occasion when you felt furious. What happened? How did you react? How did you feel physically and emotionally?
* ***Identifying Triggers:*** Reflect on the circumstances you described. What particular triggers led to your anger? Were there any trends or connections to earlier experiences?
* ***Physical and Emotional Signals:*** What bodily feelings did you observe while you were angry? How did your feelings evolve during the experience?
* ***Thought Patterns:*** What ideas were flowing through your head throughout the angry episode? Were there any negative or

critical thoughts that heightened your anger?

* ***Impact on Relationships:*** How did your anger affect your relationships with others in this situation? What were the short-term and long-term consequences?

* ***Alternative Reactions:*** Looking back, how could you have reacted differently to the situation? What methods can help you control your anger more successfully in the future?

* ***Self-Compassion:*** Write a letter to yourself showing understanding and compassion for your thoughts of rage. Acknowledge the legitimacy of your feelings and remind yourself of your commitment to handling anger productively.

You may learn more about what makes you angry and how to cope with it healthily if you use these writing prompts often. To improve your emotional health and change your relationship with anger, this self-awareness is crucial.

Chapter 5: Techniques for Managing Anger

Cognitive Restructuring

Strategies for Reframing Thoughts That Provoke Anger

Cognitive restructuring is a strong approach that helps you shift problematic cognitive processes that lead to anger. By detecting and questioning unreasonable or negative beliefs, you may replace them with more balanced and helpful ones.

Steps for Cognitive Restructuring

1. ***Identify the trigger idea:*** When you feel furious, stop and identify the particular idea that prompted your anger. This may be something like, "They never listen to me" or "This is so unfair."

2. ***Examine the evidence:*** Challenge the correctness of your thinking. Ask yourself:

- What evidence do I have that supports this thought?
- What evidence do I have that contradicts it?
- Are there any reasons for what happened?

3. ***Reframe the thought:*** Replace the negative or unreasonable thinking with a more balanced and sensible one. For example:
   - Instead of "They never listen to me," consider "Sometimes they listen, and sometimes they don't. I need to communicate more clearly."
   - Instead of "This is so unfair," try "This situation is frustrating, but I can handle it and find a solution."

4. ***Practice Empathy:*** Put yourself in the other person's shoes. Consider their viewpoint and goals. This might help you comprehend their behavior and minimize your wrath.

5. ***Use Positive Self-Talk:*** Encourage yourself with positive affirmations. For example, "I can handle this calmly" or "I am in control of my reactions."

Breathing and Relaxation Exercises

Practical Exercises to Manage Physiological Arousal:
Managing the physical signs of rage is vital for keeping your emotions in check. Breathing and relaxation techniques may help calm your nervous system and minimize physiological arousal.

Deep Breathing Exercises

1. ***Find a comfortable posture:*** Sit or lay down in a comfortable posture. Close your eyes if you feel comfortable doing so.

2. ***Inhale Slowly:*** Breathe deeply through your nose for a count of four, filling your lungs fully.

3. ***Hold Your Breath:*** Hold the breath for a count of four.

4. ***Exhale Slowly:*** Breathe out slowly through your lips for a count of six, letting all the air out.

5. ***Repeat:*** Repeat this cycle multiple times until you feel your body relaxing and your heart rate dropping.

Progressive muscle relaxation

1. ***Tighten and relax:*** Starting with your toes, tighten each muscle group in your body for five seconds, then relax. Work your way up through your legs, belly, chest, arms, and face.

2. **Focus on the release:** Pay attention to the sense of relaxation as you release the tension in each muscle area.

Visualization

1. ***Create a Calm Scene:*** Imagine yourself in a serene, tranquil area. This might be a beach, a forest, or wherever you feel comfortable and protected.

2. ***Engage Your Senses:*** Engage all your senses in this vision. Feel the sun on your skin, hear the sound of waves, and smell the fresh air.

3. ***Stay in the scenario:*** Spend a few minutes in this scenario, concentrating on your breathing and letting go of any stress.

Assertiveness Training

Skills to Express Needs and Boundaries Effectively

Being assertive implies communicating your views, emotions, and desires in a clear, honest, and courteous manner. It entails sticking up for oneself while also respecting others.

Steps for Assertiveness Training

- ***Use "I" statements:*** Express your thoughts and demands without criticizing others. For example, "I feel frustrated when I am interrupted because I lose my train of thought."

- ***Be Clear and Direct:*** Clarify what you need or desire. Avoid being ambiguous or indirect. For example, "I need quiet time to concentrate on my work."

- ***Maintain a Calm Tone:*** Speak in a calm, steady voice. Avoid raising your voice, even if you feel irritated.

- ***Practice Active Listening:*** Show that you are listening to the other person by nodding, keeping eye contact, and repeating what they've said to assure comprehension.

- ***Set Boundaries:*** Clearly outline your limitations and what you are comfortable with. For example, "I am not comfortable discussing this topic right now. Can we speak about anything else?"

- ***Say No When Needed:*** It's good to say no. Be firm but courteous. For example, "I appreciate the offer, but I can't take on another project right now."

Role-Playing Exercises

- ***Practice Scenarios:*** Role-play various situations with a buddy or in front of a mirror to practice being forceful. For example, rehearse how you would ask for a raise at work or how you would handle a buddy who has wounded your emotions.

- ***Feedback and Reflection:*** After role-playing, think about what seemed tough and what felt natural. Seek feedback from a trustworthy individual to develop your assertiveness abilities.

To learn to control your anger and express yourself constructively, try incorporating techniques like cognitive restructuring, deep breathing, and assertiveness training into your daily routine. Not only will these strategies assist you in maintaining your composure, but they will also improve your relationships and overall health.

Chapter 6: Healing and Forgiveness

Processing Anger

Releasing anger appropriately is vital for emotional well-being and sustaining successful relationships. Here are various techniques to process and release anger constructively:

Physical Activities

★ *Exercise:* Engage in physical activities like jogging, swimming, cycling, or a brisk stroll. Physical effort may assist in the release of pent-up energy and lower stress chemicals.

★ *Yoga and Stretching:* These practices combine physical activity with deep breathing and awareness, helping to soothe the mind and body.

Creative Outlets

★ *Art and Writing:* Express your anger in creative ways such as sketching, painting, or writing. Journaling about your emotions might be extremely healing.

★ ***Music:*** Playing a musical instrument, listening to music, or even dancing may be effective methods to channel and release anger.

Mindfulness & Meditation

Mindfulness Practices: Focus on the present moment via mindfulness meditation. This might help you become more aware of your emotions without getting overwhelmed by them.

Guided Imagery: Use guided imagery exercises to envision a serene location or circumstance, which may help shift your attention away from anger.

Communication:

Speak It Out: Find a trustworthy friend, family member, or therapist to talk about your anger. Sharing your emotions might bring relief and fresh insights.

Conflict Resolution: When appropriate, address the cause of your anger directly with the individual involved. Use "I" statements and active listening to encourage good discourse.

Relaxation Techniques

Deep Breathing: Practice deep breathing techniques to soothe your nervous system and minimize physical strain.

Progressive Muscle Relaxation: Tense and then slowly release each muscle group in your body to help relax and remove built-up tension.

Structured Anger Release

Angry Journals: Keep an angry notebook where you may freely express your ideas and emotions without judgment.

Letter Writing: Write a letter to the person or circumstance that got you furious. You don't have to mail it, but expressing your views in writing may be quite relieving.

Forgiveness

Forgiveness plays a significant part in recovering from previous anger and resentments. It doesn't imply endorsing or justifying destructive conduct, but rather, it requires letting go of the emotional load that anger and resentment may generate. Here are some crucial ideas concerning the importance of forgiveness:

1. Understanding Forgiveness

- *Definition:* Forgiveness is a conscious, intentional choice to relinquish sentiments of hatred or retribution against a person or group that has injured you, regardless of whether they deserve forgiveness.

- *Misconceptions:* Forgiveness is not erasing the hurt done, condoning the action, or reconciling with the perpetrator if it's not safe or suitable.

2. Benefits of Forgiveness

- ***Emotional Freedom:*** Forgiveness frees you from the emotional weight of wrath and resentment, leading to inner serenity and emotional equilibrium.

- ***Physical Health:*** Letting go of grudges and resentment may decrease stress, lower blood pressure, and enhance general physical health.

- ***Mental Health:*** Forgiveness is related to reduced levels of anxiety and sadness and greater levels of self-esteem and life satisfaction.

3. Steps to Forgiveness

- ***Acknowledge your sentiments:*** recognize and embrace your sentiments of rage and hurt. Understanding your feelings is the first step toward forgiveness.

- ***Empathize:*** Try to comprehend the viewpoint of the person who injured you. This doesn't imply you have to agree with their conduct, but empathy might help modify your viewpoint.

- ***Decide to Forgive:*** Make a deliberate choice to forgive. This choice is for your well-being, not necessarily for the benefit of the individual who injured you.

- ***Release the Anger:*** Use the skills for processing anger outlined earlier to help remove the emotional weight. Write about your experience, chat with someone you trust, or participate in activities that help you let go.

- ***Find Closure:*** Create a ritual or symbolic act that indicates letting go of the previous pain. This may be drafting a letter and then burning it, or another act that seems significant to you.

4. Practicing Self-Forgiveness

- ***Acknowledge Your faults:*** Recognize any faults or regrets you have and accept responsibility without self-condemnation.

- ***Show compassion:*** Treat yourself with the same love and empathy you would provide to a friend. Understand that everyone makes errors.

- ***Learn and develop:*** Reflect on what you've learned from the experience and how you can develop from it. Use this information to create great changes in your life.

Journaling Prompts for Forgiveness

Reflect on Anger and Hurt: Write about a moment when someone injured you. How did it make you feel? What influence has it had on your life?

Understanding the Other Perspective: Try to put yourself in the other person's shoes. What may have prompted their actions? What were they feeling at the time?

Benefits of Forgiveness: List the possible benefits of forgiving this individual. How may your life improve if you let go of your anger and resentment?

Actions for Forgiveness: Outline the actions you need to take to forgive this individual. What acts or adjustments in perspective can help you advance toward forgiveness?

Self-Forgiveness: Reflect on a circumstance when you need to forgive yourself. What did you gain from this experience? How can you be nicer to yourself going forward?

Finding peace, growing as an individual, and improving your relationships are all possible outcomes of learning to control your anger and learn to forgive.

Chapter 7: Building Sustainable Practices

Mindfulness and Meditation

Introducing Mindfulness Techniques to Cultivate Present-Moment Awareness
Mindfulness and meditation are great skills for fostering present-moment awareness and regulating anger successfully. By concentrating on the present and monitoring your thoughts and feelings without judgment, you may minimize the intensity of anger and react more calmly to triggering events.

Basic Mindfulness Techniques
1. **Mindful Breathing**
   - ***Find a Quiet Environment:*** Sit or lie down in a comfortable posture in a quiet environment.
   - ***Focus on Your Breath:*** Pay attention to your breathing. Notice the sensation of the air entering and exiting your nose, the rise and fall of your chest, or the

feeling of your belly expanding and
contracting.

- ***Count Your Breaths:*** To help keep
  attention, count each breath cycle (inhale
  and exhale) from one to 10, then start
  anew.

2. Body Scan Meditation

- ***Lie Down Comfortably:*** Lie on your
  back with your arms at your sides and
  your legs uncrossed.
- ***Scan Your Body:*** Slowly bring your
  attention to each area of your body,
  beginning with your toes and continuing
  up to your head. Notice any feelings,
  tightness, or places of discomfort.
- ***Breathe into Tension:*** If you feel
  tension or discomfort, breathe into that
  place and visualize the tension melting
  away with each exhale.

3. Mindful Observation

- ***Choose an object:*** Select a natural thing from inside your local area (a flower, bug, tree, etc.).
- ***Observe Without Judgment:*** Look at the thing as if you are viewing it for the first time. Notice every feature - the color, texture, form, and movement.
- ***Stay Present:*** If your attention wanders, softly return your concentration to the item without self-criticism.

4. Mindful Walking

- ***stroll slowly:*** Find a peaceful spot to stroll. Walk gently and carefully.
- ***Focus on Sensations:*** Pay attention to the feeling of your feet contacting the ground, the movement of your legs, and the rhythm of your breathing.
- ***Stay Present:*** Keep your concentration on the act of walking and the feelings in your body.

Creating a Support Network

A solid support network is vital for controlling anger and preserving emotional wellness. Building a network of understanding and supporting individuals may give you encouragement, guidance, and a feeling of belonging.

Steps to Create a Support Network

Identify Your Needs:

Reflect on what type of help you need. Do you need someone to speak to, someone who can provide practical guidance or someone who can help divert your anger?

Reach out to Trusted Individuals

- *Family and Friends:* Start with individuals you trust and feel comfortable with. Let them know that you are working on regulating your anger and would appreciate their support.
- *Community organizations:* Look for community organizations or support

groups that concentrate on anger management or emotional wellness. These organizations may create a feeling of community and shared experiences.

Professional Help

- ***Therapists and Counselors:*** Consider obtaining treatment from mental health specialists who can provide specialized counseling and support.
- ***Support Groups:*** Join support groups conducted by experts, which may provide organized assistance and techniques.

Online Communities

- ***Forums and Social Media Groups:*** There are various online venues where individuals share their experiences and help others control their anger. These may be beneficial, particularly if in-person assistance is not available.

Stay Connected

- ***Regular Check-Ins:*** Maintain regular communication with your support network. Schedule frequent meet-ups or check-ins to discuss your successes and difficulties.
- ***Offer Support:*** Remember that support networks are mutual. Be there for individuals in your network, providing your support and understanding.

Setting Goals

Setting specific, realistic objectives helps give direction and incentive in your path to control anger. Goals help you measure your progress and keep focused on your long-term emotional wellness.

Steps for Setting Anger Management Goals

Define Your Goals

- ❖ ***Specific:*** Clearly state what you aim to accomplish. For example, "I want to reduce the frequency of my angry outbursts at work."
- ❖ ***Measurable:*** Determine how you will quantify your progress. For instance, "I will track the number of outbursts per week."
- ❖ ***Doable:*** Set objectives that are tough yet doable. Consider your existing circumstances and what measures you can reasonably take.
- ❖ ***Relevant:*** Ensure your objectives are relevant to your overall well-being and personal progress.
- ❖ ***Time-Bound:*** Set a schedule for attaining your objectives. For example, "I aim to reduce my outbursts by 50% within three months."

Break Down Goals into Steps
- ❖ ***Small Steps:*** Break down big ambitions into smaller, doable actions. For instance, "Practice deep breathing exercises daily" or "Attend a weekly anger management class."
- ❖ ***Prioritize:*** Identify which actions are most critical and start with them.

Develop an action plan
- ❖ ***Plan Activities:*** Outline specific actions and techniques that can help you attain your objectives. For example, "Practice mindfulness meditation every morning" or "Journal about my triggers and responses weekly."
- ❖ ***Schedule:*** Incorporate these activities into your daily or weekly regimen. Set reminders to be consistent.

Monitor Your Progress
- ❖ ***Keep a Journal:*** Document your progress, noting what tactics are working and where you find problems.

❖ ***Adjust as needed:*** Be adaptable and open to modifying your goals or techniques if something isn't working. Setbacks are a regular part of the process.

Celebrate Milestones

❖ ***Acknowledge Progress:*** Celebrate your victories, no matter how minor. Recognizing your progress improves your drive and confidence.

❖ ***Reward Yourself:*** Treat yourself to something nice when you hit a milestone. This might be something simple, like a favorite pastime or a tiny present to oneself.

By adopting mindfulness and meditation techniques, developing a supportive network, and setting realistic objectives, you may successfully control anger and strive toward long-term emotional wellness. These tactics can help you remain grounded, encouraged, and inspired on your road to personal improvement and healthy relationships.

Conclusion

Empowerment

Empowerment is at the center of improving your relationship with rage. Recognizing that you have the potential to adjust your emotional reactions and how you express anger is a vital step towards personal development and better relationships.

Understanding Your Strength

- ★ *Innate Resilience:* Women exhibit enormous resilience and strength. Acknowledge the struggles you've faced and how these experiences have developed your emotional fortitude.
- ★ *Personal Agency:* Remember that you influence your responses and decisions. By making proactive efforts to regulate your anger, you are recovering your authority.

Positive Self-Perception

- ★ *Self-Compassion:* Treat oneself with love and understanding. Recognize that anger is a normal emotion and that you have the power to channel it productively.

★ ***Affirmations:*** Use positive affirmations to support your empowerment. Examples include, "I am in control of my emotions," "I can express my needs assertively," and "I have the power to transform my anger into positive action."

Role Models and Inspiration:

★ ***Inspirational Figures:*** Look to women who have effectively regulated their anger and utilized it as a catalyst for good change. Learn from their tales and methods.

★ ***Community Support:*** Surround yourself with helpful and inspiring others who promote your development and celebrate your success.

Transformative Actions

★ ***Useful Outlets:*** Channel your anger into useful pursuits such as activism, artistic endeavors, or community participation.

Use your passion to promote good change in your life and the lives of others.
★ ***Setting Boundaries:*** Empower yourself by creating and keeping healthy limits. Clear limits safeguard your well-being and strengthen your self-respect.

Continual Learning

★ ***Personal growth:*** Commit to continuing personal growth. Attend classes, read books, and participate in activities that develop your emotional intelligence and anger control abilities.
★ ***Adaptability:*** Be open to new methods and techniques. Recognize that regulating anger is a continual process, and be open to change as you learn more about yourself.

Final Thoughts

As you continue your path toward controlling anger and developing your emotional well-being, remember these crucial takeaways:

1. **Acceptance and Validation**

   Your rage is a legitimate feeling. Accepting and comprehending it is the first step towards managing it properly.

2. **Awareness and Recognition**

   Identify your anger triggers and the physical and emotional cues that precede fury. This knowledge is critical for early intervention and treatment.

3. **Healthy Expression**

   Use healthy outlets for anger, such as physical exercise, artistic expression, and conversation. Practice mindfulness and relaxation strategies to maintain serenity.

4. **Support Network**

   Build and develop a supporting network of friends, family, and professionals. Sharing your experiences and seeking help enhances your capacity to control anger.

5. Assertiveness and Boundaries

Develop assertiveness abilities to convey your wants and create limits successfully. This encourages respect and healthy relationships.

6. Forgiveness and Letting Go

Embrace forgiveness, both for others and for oneself. Letting go of previous anger and resentment frees you from emotional baggage and supports healing.

7. Continued Growth

Set realistic objectives for controlling anger and commit to continual personal improvement. Celebrate your progress and be open to learning and adaptability.

Encouragement for Continued Growth and Self-Care

Prioritize Self-Care: Make self-care a non-negotiable element of your routine. Engage in activities that foster your physical, emotional, and mental well-being.

Stay Committed: Understand that regulating anger is a constant effort. Stay devoted to your improvement, and don't be disheartened by failures. Each step forward, no matter how tiny, is progress.

Seek Joy and Balance: Balance your attempts to moderate anger with things that offer you pleasure and contentment. A balanced existence increases emotional resilience and overall happiness.

Empowering Affirmations:

"I am strong, resilient, and capable of managing my anger constructively."

"I have the power to transform my emotions and create positive change in my life."

"Every day, I grow more skilled at expressing my needs and maintaining my peace."

Final Note: Remember, this path is uniquely yours. Embrace each step with compassion and patience, knowing that your efforts are paving the path for a better, more powerful existence. Keep going ahead, and enjoy the strength and knowledge you earn along the journey.

By empowering yourself with these tactics and maintaining a commitment to self-care and personal development, you may improve your relationship with anger, leading to a more balanced, meaningful, and powerful existence.

Appendix

Workbook Section

Worksheets and Activities for Readers to Apply the Principles Discussed

<u>Worksheet 1: Identifying Anger Triggers</u>

Instructions: Reflect on recent situations where you felt angry. Identify the triggers and describe the context and your reaction.

Situation Description	Trigger(s)	Emotional Response	Physical Response	Reaction
Example: Argument with co-worker	Disrespectful comments	Frustration, hurt	Increased heart rate	Raised voice, walked away

Worksheet 2: Recognizing Physical and Emotional Signals

Instructions: Pay attention to your body's signals and emotions when you start to feel angry. Write down your observations.

Situation Description	Physical Signals	Emotional Signals
Example: Stuck in traffic	Tightness in chest	Irritation, impatience

<u>Worksheet 3: Cognitive Restructuring</u>

Instructions: Identify a recent anger-provoking thought, examine the evidence, and reframe it into a more balanced thought.

Anger-Provoking Thought	Evidence Supporting It	Evidence Against It	Reframed Thought
Example: "They never listen to me."	They interrupted me today	They listened yesterday	"Sometimes they listen, sometimes they don't. I need to communicate clearly."

<u>Worksheet 4: Breathing and Relaxation Exercises</u>

Instructions: Practice the following exercises daily and note how you feel before and after.

Date	Exercise Type	Duration	Before (Feelings)	After (Feelings)
Example: 6/15	Deep Breathing	5 minutes	Anxious, Tense	Calm, Relaxed

<u>Worksheet 5: Assertiveness Practice</u>

Instructions: Describe a situation where you need to be assertive. Write out how you will use "I" statements and set boundaries.

Situation Description	Assertive Statement (Using "I" Statements)	Boundaries Set
Example: Friend frequently cancels plans	"I feel disappointed when plans are canceled at the last minute. I need more notice."	"Please let me know at least a day in advance if plans change."

Worksheet 6: Forgiveness and Reflection

Instructions: Reflect on a situation where you need to forgive someone or yourself. Write about the impact of holding onto anger and the benefits of forgiveness.

Situation Description	Impact of Holding Onto Anger	Benefits of Forgiveness	Steps to Forgive
Example: Friend betrayed trust	Distrust and ongoing resentment	Peace of mind, improved relationship	Understanding their perspective, communicating my feelings

<u>**Worksheet 7: Goal Setting for Anger Management**</u>

Instructions: Set SMART goals for managing your anger. Break them down into actionable steps and monitor your progress.

Goal Description	Specific Steps	Timeline	Progress Tracking
Example: Reduce outbursts at work	Practice deep breathing daily, attend anger management classes, and journal triggers weekly	3 months	Weekly self-checks, progress review with therapist

Glossary

Key Terms Related to Anger and Anger Management

1. **Anger**: An emotional response characterized by feelings of irritation, frustration, and hostility towards something perceived as wrong or unjust.
2. **Anger Triggers**: Specific situations, people, or events that provoke anger.
3. **Assertiveness**: The quality of being self-assured and confident without being aggressive. It involves expressing one's needs and rights while respecting others.
4. **Cognitive Restructuring**: A therapeutic process that helps individuals identify and challenge irrational or negative thoughts, replacing them with more balanced and constructive ones.
5. **Deep Breathing**: A relaxation technique involving slow, deep inhalations and exhalations to calm the nervous system and reduce stress.

6. **Empathy**: The ability to understand and share the feelings of another person, which can help in managing anger by seeing things from another's perspective.

7. **Forgiveness**: The act of letting go of resentment and anger towards someone who has wronged you. It is a personal process that can lead to emotional healing.

8. **Mindfulness**: A mental practice focused on being fully present and aware of the moment, observing thoughts and emotions without judgment.

9. **Progressive Muscle Relaxation**: A technique that involves tensing and then slowly relaxing each muscle group in the body to reduce physical tension.

10. **Self-Awareness**: The conscious knowledge of one's character, feelings, motives, and desires, which is essential for understanding and managing anger.

11. **Self-Care**: Activities and practices that individuals engage in regularly to reduce stress and maintain and enhance their well-being and health.

12. **Support Network**: A group of people, such as friends, family, and professionals, who provide emotional and practical support.
13. **Triggers**: External events or circumstances that cause an emotional reaction, such as anger.

By utilizing these worksheets and understanding key terms, you can apply the principles discussed throughout the book to your own life, empowering yourself to manage anger constructively and foster personal growth.

www.ingramcontent.com/pod-product-compliance
Lightning Source LLC
Chambersburg PA
CBHW051840250726

48659CB00005B/1944